DIPHTHERIA DISEASE OUTBREAKS 2023

"The Silent Assassin of History: Unmasking Diphtheria's Lethal Legacy"

BY

Prof. Michael Daniel Williams

1.0 Introduction

In the annals of medical history, there exists a shadowy figure, once the scourge of childhood and the tormentor of communities. Its name, whispered with dread, is Diphtheria. In the not-so-distant past, this bacterial specter cast its sinister pall over the world, claiming the lives of countless innocents, particularly the young. It was an era when parents trembled at the mere mention of its name, when entire neighborhoods held their collective breath, and when medical science waged an unrelenting war to uncover its secrets.

Diphtheria, caused by the cunning bacterium *Corynebacterium diphtheriae*, is far more than a historical footnote. While largely subdued in many parts of the globe through vaccination and vigilant public health measures, its story is a chilling reminder of the power of infectious disease to sow terror and destruction. Yet, it is also a testament to the tenacity of humanity, as the battle against diphtheria represents one of modern medicine's most significant victories.

In this exploration, we will venture deep into the heart of this ancient adversary, dissecting its biology, unraveling its mechanisms of harm, and tracing its evolution from a ruthless killer to a managed threat. Along the way, we will uncover the importance of vaccines, the heroism of medical pioneers, and the enduring lessons that diphtheria imparts upon us a stark reminder that the specter of infectious disease is never fully vanquished but rather held at bay through knowledge, vigilance, and unwavering commitment to the preservation of life.

TABLE OF CONTENT

1.1. Historical Overview

1.2. Definition and Basic Information

2. Etiology

2.1. Corynebacterium diphtheriae: Characteristics and Classification

2.2. Toxin Production and Mechanism

3. Epidemiology

3.1. Global Prevalence and Distribution

3.2. Factors Influencing Outbreaks

4. Clinical Manifestations

4.1. Respiratory Diphtheria

4.2. Cutaneous Diphtheria

4.3. Other Forms

5.1. Clinical Examination

5.2. Laboratory Tests and Identification

6. Treatment

6.1. Antitoxin Administration

6.2. Antibiotic Therapy

6.3. Supportive Care

7. Prevention and Control

7.1. Vaccination

7.1.1. DTaP and Td Vaccines:

-Td (Tetanus and Diphtheria): Given as a booster dose to adolescents and adults every 10 years to maintain immunity. Sometimes Tdap, which includes protection against pertussis, might be given instead.

7.2. Public Health Measures

8. Complications and Prognosis

Complications:

Prognosis:

9. Recent Developments and Research

9.2. Antibiotic Resistance:

9.3. Genetic Studies:

9.4. Toxin Mechanism and Neutralization:

9.5. Epidemiological Studies:

9.6. Public Health Initiatives:

10. Conclusion and Recommendations

Conclusion:

Recommendations:

Call to Action

REFERENCE

1.1. Historical Overview

Diphtheria, known for centuries, was a leading cause of childhood mortality before the development of vaccines and antibiotics. Historical accounts date as far back as the 5th century BCE, where it was described by Hippocrates. The disease got its name from the Greek word "diphthera," which means "leather," referring to the characteristic leather-like pseudomembrane that forms in the throats of infected individuals.

1.2. Definition and Basic Information

Diphtheria is an infectious disease primarily affecting the mucous membranes of the respiratory tract (nose and throat) and occasionally the skin. It is caused by the bacterium *Corynebacterium diphtheriae*. The primary concern with diphtheria is the toxin produced by the bacterium, which can lead to serious complications, including myocarditis (heart inflammation) and neuritis (nerve inflammation).

2. Etiology

Maddie are you ok darling but now I've been very sick

2.1. *Corynebacterium diphtheriae*: Characteristics and Classification

Corynebacterium diphtheriae is a gram-positive, non-spore-forming, club-shaped bacterium. It's the primary causative agent of diphtheria. Based on biochemical and biophysical properties, this bacterium is divided into four biotypes: gravis, mitis, intermedius, and belfanti.

Among these, the gravis and mitis biotypes are most frequently associated with human infections.

2.2. Toxin Production and Mechanism

The virulence of *Corynebacterium diphtheriae* primarily stems from its ability to produce an exotoxin known as diphtheria toxin. This toxin is the result of the bacterium being infected by a bacteriophage (a virus that infects bacteria) carrying the toxin gene.

Once the toxin enters the host's cells, it inhibits protein synthesis, leading to cell death. The severity of diphtheria is often linked to the amount of toxin produced and dispersed throughout the body. The toxin primarily targets the heart, nerves, and kidneys. Its effects can lead to potentially fatal complications if not treated promptly.

It's worth noting that not all strains of *Corynebacterium diphtheriae* produce toxins. Only those that are lysogenized by a specific bacteriophage can produce the diphtheria toxin.

3. Epidemiology

3.1. Global Prevalence and Distribution

Historically, diphtheria was a major health concern worldwide, causing numerous deaths, particularly among children. The introduction of the diphtheria vaccine led to a significant decline in cases in developed countries. However, in regions with low vaccination rates or interrupted immunization services, diphtheria remains a concern.

During the 1990s, a major outbreak occurred in the former Soviet Union, illustrating the disease's potential to return if public health measures are not maintained.

As of the last data before 2021, the World Health Organization reported sporadic cases in various regions, with larger outbreaks occurring in countries with suboptimal vaccination coverage.

3.2. Factors Influencing Outbreaks

Several factors can contribute to the emergence or re-emergence of diphtheria:

- **Vaccination Coverage**: The primary defense against diphtheria is vaccination. Areas with low vaccination rates are vulnerable to outbreaks.

- **Population Movement**: Migration or the movement of non-immunized individuals into an area can introduce the disease.

- **Healthcare Infrastructure**: Weak health systems, lack of surveillance, and inadequate treatment facilities can exacerbate the spread.

- **Socioeconomic Factors**: Poverty, limited access to healthcare, and lack of education can contribute to reduced vaccination rates and increased susceptibility.

- **Environmental Factors**: Overcrowding and poor sanitation can facilitate the spread of respiratory diseases, including diphtheria.

4. Clinical Manifestations

4.1. Respiratory Diphtheria

Respiratory diphtheria primarily affects the nasopharynx and tonsils. Initial symptoms resemble a common cold, including:

- Mild fever
- Sore throat
- Fatigue
- Swollen glands

As the disease progresses, a distinguishing feature of diphtheria emerges: the formation of a thick, gray or white pseudomembrane covering the tonsils and throat. This pseudomembrane is firm and can cause difficulty breathing or swallowing. It can be potentially life-threatening if it obstructs the airway.

4.2. Cutaneous Diphtheria

While less common than respiratory diphtheria, *Corynebacterium diphtheriae* can also infect skin wounds, leading to cutaneous diphtheria. Symptoms include:

- Non-healing ulcers with a grayish membrane
- Surrounding skin may be swollen and red

This form of diphtheria is more common in tropical areas and among those with compromised skin integrity, like individuals with eczema or skin injuries.

4.3. Other Forms

In rare cases, diphtheria can affect other parts of the body:

- **Ocular Diphtheria**: Involves the eye, leading to symptoms like pain, redness, discharge, and formation of a membrane on the conjunctiva.

- **Laryngeal Diphtheria**: Affects the voice box, causing hoarseness, cough, and potential airway obstruction.

- **Nasal Diphtheria**: Causes a nasal discharge and formation of a membrane in the nasal passages.

5. Diagnosis

5.1. Clinical Examination

A preliminary diagnosis of diphtheria is often based on clinical presentation. The presence of a characteristic pseudomembrane in the throat, especially in a patient with a sore throat and fever, can raise suspicions of diphtheria. It's essential to differentiate diphtheria from other conditions like tonsillitis, pharyngitis, and mononucleosis that can have similar symptoms but different treatments.

5.2. Laboratory Tests and Identification

Definitive diagnosis requires laboratory confirmation:

- **Culture**: A swab from the patient's throat or nose, or from a skin lesion in the case of cutaneous diphtheria, is taken and cultured on a special medium called Loeffler's medium or Tinsdale agar. The growth of *Corynebacterium diphtheriae* on this medium can help confirm the diagnosis.

- **Toxin Testing**: Since not all strains of *Corynebacterium diphtheriae* produce the diphtheria toxin, it's crucial to test for toxin production. The Elek test is a common method for detecting diphtheria toxin.

- **Gram Stain**: A Gram stain of the specimen can be done to visualize the characteristic morphology of the bacteria.

- **PCR**: Polymerase chain reaction (PCR) can be used to identify the bacteria and detect the toxin gene, providing rapid and accurate results.

6. Treatment

Treating diphtheria effectively requires a combination of neutralizing the toxin and eradicating the causative bacterium. Here's how this is achieved:

6.1. Antitoxin Administration

Diphtheria antitoxin, derived from hyperimmunized horses, is the primary treatment for diphtheria toxin. It neutralizes the toxin circulating in the bloodstream. The antitoxin doesn't neutralize toxin that is already bound to tissues, so early administration is crucial to prevent complications. Before administration, a skin test may be done to check for potential allergic reactions, though in emergency situations, this step might be skipped due to the life-saving nature of the antitoxin.

6.2. Antibiotic Therapy

Antibiotics are given to eradicate the *Corynebacterium diphtheriae* bacterium and prevent its transmission to others. Commonly used antibiotics include:

-Erythromycin: Given orally or by injection.

-Penicillin: Administered by injection for those not allergic to penicillin.

Even after symptoms have resolved, patients are typically kept in isolation until they have completed antibiotic treatment to prevent spreading the bacterium to others. Follow-up throat swabs may be taken to confirm the bacterium's absence.

6.3. Supportive Care

In addition to specific treatments, supportive care is essential, especially for patients with severe symptoms. This might include:

-**Hospitalization**: Especially if there's difficulty breathing or severe complications.

-**Oxygen therapy**: For patients with respiratory distress.

-**Intravenous fluids**: To maintain hydration if swallowing is difficult.

-**Airway management**: In extreme cases where the pseudomembrane obstructs breathing, intubation or a tracheostomy might be required.

7. Prevention and Control

Diphtheria is a preventable disease, and several measures can be employed to control its spread and prevent outbreaks.

7.1. Vaccination

Vaccination is the primary method of diphtheria prevention.

7.1.1. DTaP and Td Vaccines:

-DTaP (Diphtheria, Tetanus, and Pertussis): This vaccine is given to children in multiple doses, typically at ages 2, 4, 6, and

15-18 months, and then again between 4-6 years.

-Td (Tetanus and Diphtheria):

Given as a booster dose to adolescents and adults every 10 years to maintain immunity. Sometimes Tdap, which includes protection against pertussis, might be given instead.

7.1.2. Schedule and Dosage:

Regular boosters are essential because immunity to diphtheria decreases over time. Adults should ensure they're up-to-date with their boosters, especially if traveling to areas where diphtheria is prevalent.

7.2. Public Health Measures

i. Surveillance and Reporting: Timely reporting of suspected cases allows for rapid response and containment. Effective surveillance systems can detect and respond to outbreaks early.

ii. Quarantine and Isolation: Patients diagnosed with diphtheria are typically isolated until they're no longer contagious. This can prevent the spread of the bacterium to others.

iii. Contact Tracing and Prophylaxis: People who have been in close contact with someone diagnosed with diphtheria should be identified. They may be given a dose of antibiotics to prevent the development of the disease and may also need a booster vaccine if their immunizations are not up-to-date.

iv. Education and Awareness: Public health campaigns can inform communities about the importance of vaccination and early symptoms of diphtheria. This is particularly vital in areas with low vaccination rates.

8. Complications and Prognosis

Diphtheria, if not treated promptly, can lead to serious complications due to the toxin's effect on various body systems. Here are the major complications associated with diphtheria:

Complications:

a. **Myocarditis (Heart inflammation):** The diphtheria toxin can damage the heart muscle, leading to symptoms like shortness of breath, rapid heartbeat, and chest pain. In severe cases, myocarditis can lead to heart failure.

b. **Neuritis (Nerve inflammation):** Several weeks after the onset of diphtheria, some patients can develop neuritis. This might manifest as blurred or double vision, difficulty swallowing, and slurred speech. Eventually, it can progress to nerve damage, leading to paralysis in some parts of the body.

c. **Airway obstruction:**
The pseudomembrane formed in the throat can become thick and large enough to block the airway, leading to breathing difficulties and potential suffocation.

d. **Secondary bacterial infections:**
The presence of the pseudomembrane and tissue damage can predispose individuals to secondary bacterial infections like pneumonia.

e. **Kidney damage:** The diphtheria toxin can lead to inflammation and damage to the kidneys, impairing their function.

f. **Septicemia:** In rare cases, the bacteria can enter the bloodstream and cause a widespread infection, leading to septicemia or blood poisoning.

Prognosis:

With early diagnosis and appropriate treatment, most patients recover fully from diphtheria. However, the delay in treatment can increase the risk of serious complications. The case fatality rate for diphtheria varies:

- With treatment, the fatality rate is between 5-10%.

- Without adequate treatment, the fatality rate can be as high as 20% or more, especially in vulnerable populations like young children and the elderly.

9. Recent Developments and Research

As of my last update in September 2021, the focus on diphtheria had largely been on prevention through vaccination, early detection, and prompt treatment. However, like many infectious diseases, continuous research and developments are being carried out to enhance our understanding and management of the disease. Here's a general overview of areas of interest and potential developments:

9.1. Vaccine Development and Enhancement:

While the current diphtheria vaccine is effective, research is ongoing to improve vaccine formulations, enhance immunogenicity, and potentially lengthen the duration of immunity.

9.2. Antibiotic Resistance:

With the rising global concern over antibiotic resistance, studies are underway to monitor strains of *Corynebacterium diphtheriae* for resistance to common antibiotics. This knowledge would guide treatment protocols and potentially lead to the development of new drugs.

9.3. Genetic Studies:

Advances in genomic technologies provide insights into the genetic makeup of the diphtheria bacterium. These studies can help in understanding pathogenicity, transmission patterns, and potentially identifying new therapeutic targets.

9.4. Toxin Mechanism and Neutralization:

Further exploration of the diphtheria toxin's mechanism of action and its interactions with host cells might lead to the development of novel antitoxin therapies or enhance the effectiveness of current treatments.

9.5. Epidemiological Studies:

Given the sporadic outbreaks of diphtheria in various parts of the world, studies focusing on the disease's epidemiology can help in understanding transmission dynamics, identifying high-risk populations, and implementing targeted public health measures.

9.6. Public Health Initiatives:

Research into the socio-economic and cultural factors affecting vaccine uptake can inform public health campaigns, ensuring that they are culturally sensitive and effective in increasing immunization rates.

10. Conclusion and Recommendations

Conclusion:

Diphtheria, once a major cause of illness and death worldwide, has seen a significant decline in prevalence thanks to extensive vaccination campaigns and public health measures. While it remains controlled in many parts of the world, sporadic outbreaks and cases emphasize the continuous need for vigilance. Its potential severity, coupled with the ease of prevention through vaccination, necessitates ongoing efforts to ensure global control and, eventually, eradication.

Recommendations:

1. **Strengthen Vaccination Campaigns**: Sustain high vaccination rates by conducting regular immunization drives, especially in areas with historically low coverage.

2. **Educate and Raise Awareness**: Continuous public health awareness campaigns highlighting the importance of vaccination, recognizing early symptoms, and seeking prompt medical attention.

3. **Surveillance and Rapid Response**: Establish and maintain robust disease surveillance systems to detect and respond to outbreaks promptly. Quick identification and containment can prevent widespread transmission.

4. **Research and Development**: Continued investment in research to

enhance vaccines, understand antibiotic resistance patterns, and explore new treatment modalities.

5. **International Collaboration**: Collaborative efforts between countries can facilitate the sharing of best practices, resources, and data. This can be particularly effective in managing diseases that know no borders.

6. **Ensure Access**: Making vaccines and treatments affordable and accessible to all, regardless of socio-economic status, is crucial for widespread protection.

7. **Periodic Review**: Periodically review and update guidelines and recommendations based on new research and findings to ensure that the best preventive and therapeutic measures are in place.

Call to Action

In an age where information is at our fingertips and scientific advancements are made daily, complacency is our greatest enemy. We must remain steadfast, ensuring that every child is vaccinated, every community educated, and every individual remains vigilant. The fight against diphtheria is not just a battle of the past—it's a continuous journey towards safeguarding our future. Join the crusade. Be the sentinel against resurgence. Advocate, educate, and vaccinate, because history, as we've so painfully learned, should never be allowed to repeat itself. Act now. The legacy of tomorrow depends on the choices we make today.

REFERENCE

1. **World Health Organization (WHO)**

- Title: "Diphtheria"- Link:

https://www.who.int/health-topics/diphtheria/about

- Description: An overview of diphtheria, its epidemiology, prevention, and control measures.

2. **Centers for Disease Control and Prevention (CDC)**

- Title: "Diphtheria"- Link:

https://www.cdc.gov/diphtheria/index.html

- Description: Provides details about symptoms, transmission, and prevention of diphtheria.

3. Medscape

-Title:"DiphtheriaClinical Presentation"-Link:

https://emedicine.medscape.com/article/782051-clinical

- Description: A detailed review of the clinical aspects of diphtheria.

4. Textbooks:

- "Harrison's Principles of Internal Medicine" - This foundational medical textbook offers information on a vast array of diseases, including diphtheria.

- "Mandell, Douglas, and Bennett's Principles and Practice of Infectious Diseases" - Provides in-depth information about various infectious diseases.

5. Research Journals:

- A search on PubMed or Google Scholar using the keyword "diphtheria" would provide numerous research articles, reviews, and case studies that can serve as references.

CONTENTS

Title Page

Disclaimer   1

Daily Menu and Regime   3

Sleep Position   6

Corn   7

Coffee   9

Coffee With Milk   11

Cheese   13

Avocado   15

Mortadella   17

Blood Sausage   19

Aguamiel   21

Chocolate   23

Vitamin Drink   25

Rice   27

Pasta   29

Sweet Potato   31

Chicken   33

Beef   35

Honeydew Melon   37

Papaya   38

Oats   39

Banana   40

Hygiene   41

5 Meals a Day   42

Alcohol   44

Uric Acid Medicine   45

Going to Bed Early   46

Some Thoughts   48

DISCLAIMER

The information presented in this book is intended for general informational purposes only and should not be considered a substitute for professional medical advice, diagnosis, or treatment. The content provided is based on the experiences and perspectives of the featured 114-year-old individual and should be viewed as anecdotal and not as medical or scientific fact.

It is important to consult with a qualified healthcare professional or medical expert before making any significant changes to your lifestyle, including dietary habits, exercise routines, or other health-related choices. Longevity and health are complex subjects, and individual needs and circumstances may vary greatly. What works for one person may not be suitable for another.

The author and publisher of this book do not endorse or guarantee the effectiveness of any specific longevity advice or practices mentioned within its pages. Any actions taken based on the information presented are at the reader's own risk.

Furthermore, the 114-year-old man's unique life experiences and choices may not be representative of the general population's experiences with aging and longevity. His story is intended to inspire and offer insight, but it should not be considered a blueprint for achieving a long and healthy life.

Readers are encouraged to conduct their own research, seek guidance from medical professionals, and consider their own health conditions and individual circumstances when making decisions about their well-being. The author and publisher disclaim any liability or responsibility for any consequences resulting from the use of the information in this book.

The author generated some of the text in part with GPT-3.5, OpenAI's large-scale language-generation model. Upon generating draft language, the author reviewed, edited, and revised the language to their own liking and takes ultimate responsibility for the content of this publication.

DAILY MENU AND REGIME

The daily menu and regime described serve as a general framework and should be adjusted under unique circumstances. They should be considered as guidelines rather than strict rules, and should be adjusted as needed.

Food to eat and beverage to drink
Easy to chew
Easy to digest
The food and beverage doesn't make the stomach upset.

Before 6 AM
Wakes up
Stays in bed until breakfast is ready

8:30 AM
Breakfast
Light and not too heavy
Arepa with corn flour
Cheese, avocado, mortadella, even blood sausage.
Coffee with or without whole fat milk or aguamiel (it's a kind of tea made with water and panela, the latter a derivative of sugarcane). Generally the coffee is without milk.

10-10:30 AM
Snack
Sandwich
Biscuits
Pancakes

Milk chocolate to eat
Dark chocolate to drink
Ensure vitamin drink, Sustagen vitamin drink or any other vitamin drink
Water or aguamiel (it's a kind of tea made with water and panela, the latter a derivative of sugarcane)

1 PM
Lunch
Largest meal
White rice
White pasta
Sweet potato
Very soft meat
Chicken
Soft beef or ground beef. Little beef due to uric acid
Fish (brague, tuna, sardines). No seafood because it is very expensive

Vegetable soup. Very little tomatoes due to uric acid
Avocado
Unripe bananas
Cakes
Hallacas
Mondongo (soup)
Honey water or juice of any fruit. The fruit is mostly melon and papaya. The type of melon is typically honeydew melon.

3 PM
Snack
Biscuits, pancakes, chocolate to eat or drink, Ensure vitamins drink or Sustagen vitamins drink
Water or aguamiel (it's a kind of tea made with water and panela, the latter a derivative of sugarcane)

5:30 PM
Dinner

Light meal
Bread with cheese or just bread with a drink or porridge (Oats, maizena (corn starch), banana).
Empanadas
Water or coffee with or without whole fat milk. Generally the coffee is without milk.

After dinner
Goes to bed

Beverage
Mostly water, honey water, coffee, and wine. Rarely a dark chocolate drink. When Juan Vicente Perez Mora was younger, he drank liquor and michito.

Candy
Soft caramels
Chocolate

Eats little
Beans and lentils as it can upset his stomach.
Mayonnaise and ketchup
Tomates
Meat

Eats/drinks rarely
Carbonated water and soda
Burger and pizza
Fried food
Fast food

Avoid
Nuts
Hazelnut cocoa spread
Champignon and mushrooms
Energy drinks
Pickled vegetables
Very spicy food

SLEEP POSITION

In Juan Vicente Pérez Mora's fascinating journey to a long and healthy life, his diverse sleeping habits - alternating between the right side, left side, and occasionally on his back - have been part of his routine. While the direct link between these sleeping positions and an extended lifespan remains unverified, understanding the potential benefits associated with each position sheds light on their impact on overall well-being and quality of sleep.

Sleeping on the right side, for instance, can help alleviate symptoms related to acid reflux and heartburn. By positioning the body in this way, the pressure on the stomach is reduced, minimizing the potential for stomach acid to flow back into the esophagus. This could contribute to a more comfortable night's rest and alleviate discomfort caused by digestive issues, indirectly promoting better sleep quality.

Conversely, sleeping on the left side can be beneficial for certain individuals, particularly those dealing with heart conditions. This position allows the heart to pump more efficiently due to the heart's natural orientation within the chest. It enhances circulation and reduces potential strain on the heart, potentially leading to better rest and improved cardiac health.

Occasionally, sleeping on the back, while not the primary position, might aid in reducing snoring or addressing mild sleep apnea. This position helps keep the airways more open, reducing the occurrence of obstructive breathing patterns during sleep and leading to a more restful night.

CORN

Corn is a versatile and nutrient-rich grain. It's a good source of various essential nutrients, including fiber, vitamins, and minerals. Its nutritional profile makes it a valuable addition to a well-rounded diet, which can positively impact health and, over time, potentially contribute to longevity.

One of the primary advantages of corn is its high fiber content. Fiber is essential for digestive health, aiding in regular bowel movements and supporting the growth of beneficial gut bacteria. A healthy digestive system is crucial for nutrient absorption and overall well-being. The fiber in corn can also help lower cholesterol levels, potentially reducing the risk of heart disease, a leading cause of mortality.

Corn is a significant source of antioxidants, including carotenoids like lutein and zeaxanthin. These compounds are essential for eye health and may help reduce the risk of age-related macular degeneration, a leading cause of vision loss in older adults. By supporting eye health, corn's antioxidants contribute to a higher quality of life as one ages.

Moreover, corn contains essential vitamins and minerals. It's a good source of thiamine (vitamin B1), which plays a vital role in nerve function and energy metabolism. Niacin (vitamin B3) found in corn is crucial for the conversion of food into energy. The mineral phosphorus, also abundant in corn, is necessary for bone health and energy production.

Additionally, corn is a source of carbohydrates, offering sustained energy. The complex carbohydrates in corn release energy gradually, aiding in maintaining stable blood sugar levels. Stable blood sugar is crucial in preventing energy crashes and mood fluctuations, promoting a consistent and healthy lifestyle.

Corn also contains small amounts of protein and healthy fats. While not a primary source of protein, the combination of amino acids in corn contributes to the body's overall protein intake, supporting various bodily functions and tissues.

The diverse applications of corn in various cuisines worldwide allow for creative and healthy meal choices. It can be incorporated into numerous dishes, from salads to soups and even ground into cornmeal for baking or cooking.

However, while corn offers numerous health benefits, it's essential to consume it as part of a balanced diet. Relying solely on one food, even one as nutritious as corn, may not provide all the necessary nutrients for optimal health. Variety in diet is key to ensuring the intake of a wide range of essential nutrients.

COFFEE

Coffee, one of the world's most beloved beverages, has been extensively studied for its potential health benefits, and its consumption has been associated with various positive effects that might contribute to a healthier and potentially longer life.

The most well-known component of coffee is caffeine, a natural stimulant that can enhance cognitive function, increase alertness, and improve mood. Caffeine blocks an inhibitory neurotransmitter in the brain, leading to a stimulant effect that can enhance various aspects of brain function, such as memory, mood, and reaction time.

Moreover, coffee is rich in antioxidants. These compounds help combat oxidative stress in the body, which can contribute to the aging process and various chronic diseases. Antioxidants in coffee, like chlorogenic acid, may help protect cells from damage caused by free radicals.

Regular, moderate coffee consumption has been associated with a reduced risk of certain diseases. Studies suggest that moderate coffee intake may lower the risk of developing type 2 diabetes. The compounds in coffee can improve insulin sensitivity, regulate blood sugar levels, and decrease inflammation, all of which are crucial factors in preventing diabetes.

Additionally, research has shown that coffee consumption may lower the risk of certain types of cancer, such as liver and colorectal cancer. The compounds present in coffee, including polyphenols and antioxidants, exhibit potential anti-carcinogenic properties, aiding in the prevention of cell damage and abnormal cell growth.

Notably, coffee has also been linked to a reduced risk of neurodegenerative diseases like Alzheimer's and Parkinson's. The caffeine and antioxidants in coffee may protect the brain by suppressing the production of proteins associated with these conditions and reducing the risk of cognitive decline.

Moderate coffee consumption—generally up to two cups a day—has also been associated with a lower risk of stroke and certain heart conditions. The antioxidants in coffee might help improve blood vessel function and decrease inflammation, positively impacting cardiovascular health.

However, consuming more than two cups of coffee daily might lead to adverse effects such as increased heart rate, anxiety, and disrupted sleep. Additionally, excessive coffee intake can increase the risk of stomach pain, as the acidic nature of coffee may cause discomfort in some individuals.

In conclusion, while coffee consumption has shown various potential health benefits, it's important to consume it in moderation and as part of a balanced diet. Coffee's antioxidants, caffeine, and other compounds may contribute to a healthier lifestyle when combined with other healthy habits such as a balanced diet and regular exercise. Moderation is key to enjoying the potential benefits of coffee while minimizing potential adverse effects.

COFFEE WITH MILK

Coffee, when mixed with milk, retains many of its own health advantages. The beverage's high antioxidant content remains unchanged, offering protection against oxidative stress and potentially reducing the risk of certain diseases. These antioxidants in coffee combined with the nutrients in milk create a powerful, synergistic effect that can positively impact overall health.

The addition of milk to coffee can provide essential nutrients that coffee alone might lack. Milk is a significant source of calcium, vital for maintaining strong bones and teeth. This combination can be especially beneficial for individuals looking to increase their calcium intake without relying solely on dairy products.

Furthermore, milk contains protein, an essential component for muscle repair and growth, making coffee with milk a good option for a post-workout beverage. This combination offers a balance of carbohydrates, protein, and caffeine, aiding in post-exercise recovery and providing an energy boost.

The mixture of coffee and milk may also address some of the potential adverse effects associated with drinking coffee alone. For instance, combining coffee with milk might help alleviate issues like acidity and digestive discomfort that some individuals experience when consuming coffee on an empty stomach. The milk's proteins may help neutralize some of the acidic properties of coffee, reducing the likelihood of stomach irritation.

The pairing of coffee with milk also provides a more balanced and satiating drink. The protein and fat content in milk can slow down the absorption of caffeine, resulting in a more gradual and prolonged energy boost compared to drinking black coffee. This steadier release of caffeine into the bloodstream might reduce the likelihood of the jittery feeling sometimes associated with coffee consumption.

However, it's important to note that the health benefits of coffee with milk can be influenced by the type and quantity of milk used. Whole milk, for instance, provides more fat and calories than low-fat or plant-based milk alternatives. Careful consideration should be given to individual dietary preferences and health goals when choosing the type of milk used in coffee.

In summary, combining coffee with milk presents a marriage of coffee's antioxidants and milk's nutrients, potentially offering a diverse range of health benefits. This combination can provide a more balanced, satisfying beverage, making it an appealing choice for individuals seeking the advantages of both coffee and milk in a single, versatile drink.

CHEESE

Cheese, a rich and diverse dairy product, contributes several nutritional benefits that, when consumed as part of a balanced diet, can positively impact overall health and potentially support a longer and healthier life.

Cheese is a concentrated source of several vital nutrients. It's abundant in calcium, a crucial mineral necessary for strong bones and teeth. Regular consumption of cheese can aid in meeting the body's calcium requirements, especially for individuals who might have difficulty obtaining adequate amounts from other sources.

Moreover, cheese is a source of high-quality protein, essential for various bodily functions such as muscle repair, growth, and overall health maintenance. Protein from cheese can be particularly beneficial for vegetarians and individuals seeking alternative sources of protein in their diet.

The fermentation process involved in cheese production can lead to the formation of probiotics. These beneficial bacteria, found in certain types of cheese like yogurt or aged varieties, contribute to gut health by promoting a balanced gut microbiome. A healthy gut environment is associated with improved digestion, better nutrient absorption, and enhanced immune function.

Additionally, cheese contains various essential vitamins, such as vitamin A, B vitamins (including B12), and vitamin K2. Vitamin A is essential for vision and a robust immune system, while B vitamins play a role in energy production and brain function. Vitamin K2 is crucial for bone health, aiding in calcium metabolism and deposition in bones.

The fat content in cheese, while varying among different types, may contribute to satiety and provide a concentrated source of energy. However, it's important to consume cheese in moderation, especially for individuals watching their overall fat intake, as some varieties can be high in saturated fats.

The rich flavors and textures of cheese can add diversity to the diet, making it an enjoyable addition to various meals. Whether incorporated into sandwiches, salads, or paired with fruits and nuts, cheese offers a versatile and flavorful option for enhancing the nutritional value of dishes.

Though cheese offers numerous health benefits, its consumption should be part of a balanced diet. While it provides essential nutrients, excessive intake can contribute to high saturated fat and sodium levels, potentially increasing the risk of certain health conditions such as heart disease or high blood pressure.

In conclusion, cheese's nutritional profile includes a variety of essential nutrients and beneficial components, making it a valuable addition to a balanced diet when consumed in moderation. When paired with a variety of other nutritious foods, cheese can contribute to overall health and well-being, potentially supporting a longer and healthier life.

AVOCADO

Avocado, a unique and nutrient-rich fruit, provides a myriad of health benefits that, when incorporated into a balanced diet, can contribute to improved overall health and potentially support a longer and healthier life.

One of the primary advantages of avocados is their healthy fat content. They are a rich source of monounsaturated fats, particularly oleic acid. These healthy fats are known to support heart health by reducing bad cholesterol levels and increasing good cholesterol, helping to maintain a healthy cardiovascular system and lower the risk of heart disease.

Moreover, avocados are a good source of dietary fiber. High fiber content contributes to improved digestion and aids in maintaining a healthy weight by promoting feelings of fullness. The fiber in avocados also supports gut health, benefiting the balance of the gut microbiome and aiding in the prevention of certain digestive issues.

The fruit is also abundant in various vitamins and minerals. Avocados contain essential nutrients such as potassium, which is crucial for maintaining healthy blood pressure levels and proper muscle function. They also provide vitamins C, E, K, and various B vitamins, which play a role in immune function, skin health, and energy metabolism.

Furthermore, avocados contain antioxidants, such as carotenoids and tocopherols, which help combat oxidative stress and inflammation in the body. These antioxidants contribute to overall health by reducing the risk of chronic diseases and supporting healthy aging.

The unique combination of healthy fats, fiber, and a wide array of vitamins and minerals in avocados makes them a versatile addition to a balanced diet. Whether sliced on toast, added to salads, or blended into smoothies, avocados offer a creamy texture and a delicious flavor while providing a nutrient-dense boost to meals.

While avocados offer numerous health benefits, it's important to consume them as part of a varied and balanced diet. While the fruit provides essential nutrients, excessive consumption could contribute to an excessive calorie intake, which might be a concern for individuals aiming to manage their weight.

In conclusion, avocados' nutritional richness, comprising healthy fats, fiber, antioxidants, and a range of essential vitamins and minerals, makes them a valuable addition to a healthy diet. When incorporated as part of a well-rounded eating plan, avocados can contribute to improved overall health and potentially support a longer and healthier life.

MORTADELLA

Mortadella is a type of Italian cold cut, known for its distinctive flavor and texture. While it may offer certain nutritional benefits, it's important to consider its consumption as part of a balanced diet due to its specific composition.

Mortadella is primarily made from finely ground pork, seasoned with various spices and often containing small cubes of pork fat. While it provides protein, vitamins, and minerals, it's also relatively high in saturated fat and sodium, which can be a concern for those monitoring their intake of these nutrients.

The protein content in mortadella is beneficial for muscle maintenance and repair. It contributes to a feeling of fullness and can aid in supporting a balanced diet. Mortadella also contains B vitamins, including B12 and niacin, which are essential for energy metabolism and overall well-being.

On the downside, mortadella's high sodium content might pose a challenge for individuals looking to manage their blood pressure or reduce sodium intake. Excessive sodium consumption can contribute to increased blood pressure and potentially impact heart health.

The presence of saturated fat in mortadella, primarily from the added fat, might be a concern for those aiming to control their intake of unhealthy fats. High saturated fat intake can contribute to an increased risk of heart disease and other health issues.

While mortadella can be enjoyed as part of a sandwich or in various recipes, it's important to consume it in moderation. As with many processed meats, regular and excessive consumption might increase the risk of certain health conditions and should be part of an overall balanced diet rich in fruits, vegetables, whole grains, and lean protein sources.

In conclusion, while mortadella offers some nutritional benefits such as protein and essential vitamins, its high sodium and saturated fat content should be taken into consideration. Consuming mortadella in moderation, as part of a well-rounded diet, can help individuals enjoy its flavor and unique characteristics without significantly impacting their overall health.

BLOOD SAUSAGE

Blood sausage, also known as black pudding, is a type of sausage made by cooking animal blood with various ingredients, typically grains, fats, and spices. While it does contain certain nutrients, it's important to consider its consumption within the context of its nutritional content.

Blood sausage contains iron, an essential mineral crucial for the transportation of oxygen in the body. Animal blood, a primary component of blood sausage, is rich in heme iron, which is more easily absorbed by the body compared to non-heme iron found in plant-based sources. Iron is vital for preventing anemia and maintaining overall health.

Furthermore, blood sausage often contains animal fats and proteins. These fats can provide energy and contribute to the taste and texture of the sausage. The proteins in blood sausage can aid in various bodily functions, including muscle repair and immune support.

However, blood sausage, like other processed meats, can have potential health concerns. It's typically high in saturated fat and cholesterol, which, when consumed in excess, can increase the risk of heart disease and other cardiovascular issues. Additionally, the high sodium content in some variations of blood sausage might be a concern for those managing their blood pressure or sodium intake.

It's essential to consume blood sausage in moderation due to its specific nutritional profile. While it does offer certain nutrients like iron and proteins, the potential risks associated with its high saturated fat, cholesterol, and sodium content should be taken into consideration.

In conclusion, while blood sausage contains beneficial nutrients such as heme iron and proteins, its high levels of saturated fat, cholesterol, and sodium need to be carefully managed. Enjoying blood sausage in moderation, as part of a varied and balanced diet, allows individuals to appreciate its taste while being mindful of potential health considerations.

AGUAMIEL

Aguamiel, a traditional beverage, is a sweet, sap-like liquid extracted from the agave plant. While aguamiel contains certain nutrients and has cultural significance, it's important to understand its nutritional value and consider it as part of a balanced diet.

Aguamiel is high in fructose, a natural sugar found in many fruits and honey. This natural sweetness provides energy and can be a source of carbohydrates. However, due to its high sugar content, excessive consumption of aguamiel may contribute to an increased intake of simple sugars, potentially affecting blood sugar levels.

The beverage also contains trace amounts of vitamins and minerals such as calcium, potassium, and magnesium. While these nutrients are present, they are not present in high enough quantities to significantly impact one's overall nutritional intake.

Traditionally, aguamiel has been consumed for its potential medicinal and nutritional benefits. It's believed to have hydrating properties and is sometimes used to make pulque, a fermented alcoholic beverage. The sugars in aguamiel provide a substrate for fermentation, resulting in the production of pulque.

It's important to note that while aguamiel might offer certain nutrients and cultural significance, its high sugar content should be consumed in moderation. Excessive intake of sweetened beverages, including aguamiel, may contribute to an increased risk of dental issues, weight gain, and potentially affect blood sugar regulation.

In summary, aguamiel, with its natural sugars and trace nutrients, may have cultural significance and provide some nutritional value. However, it should be consumed in moderation due to its high sugar content, and individuals should consider its role within the context of a balanced diet.

CHOCOLATE

Chocolate, derived from the cacao bean, is celebrated for its rich taste and potential health benefits when consumed in moderation as part of a balanced diet.

Dark chocolate, in particular, is known for its higher cocoa content and beneficial antioxidants. These antioxidants, such as flavonoids and polyphenols, may help reduce inflammation in the body and combat oxidative stress, potentially contributing to heart health and reducing the risk of certain diseases.

Cocoa contains compounds that have been associated with improved cardiovascular health. Consuming moderate amounts of dark chocolate has been linked to potential benefits such as reducing blood pressure and improving blood flow, contributing to overall heart health.

Additionally, dark chocolate may have a positive impact on brain function. It contains substances that may improve cognitive function and mood by increasing blood flow to the brain, potentially aiding in short-term cognitive performance and supporting overall mental well-being.

Moreover, chocolate contains minerals such as iron, magnesium, and copper, albeit in smaller quantities. While these minerals are present, they may not significantly impact one's overall nutrient intake.

However, it's important to note that chocolate also contains sugar and fat. Consuming large quantities of chocolate, particularly milk chocolate or those with added sugar and fats, may lead to excessive calorie intake and weight gain, potentially increasing the risk of health issues such as obesity and dental problems.

Enjoying chocolate in moderation is key. Opting for dark chocolate with higher cocoa content and lower added sugars can provide potential health benefits while limiting the adverse effects associated with excessive sugar and fat intake.

In conclusion, dark chocolate, especially those with higher cocoa content, offers antioxidants and potential health benefits when consumed in moderation. However, individuals should be mindful of the sugar and fat content in certain varieties of chocolate and incorporate it as part of a balanced diet to maximize its potential health benefits.

VITAMIN DRINK

Vitamin drinks, often marketed as beverages fortified with essential vitamins and minerals, can offer certain nutritional benefits. However, it's crucial to understand their composition and consider their role as part of a balanced diet.

These drinks usually contain a combination of vitamins and minerals, offering an easy way to supplement one's nutrient intake. They typically include vitamin C, B vitamins, and minerals like calcium and magnesium. Such added nutrients can be beneficial, especially for individuals with dietary deficiencies or those seeking a convenient way to increase their vitamin intake.

Vitamin drinks often cater to specific health needs. Some are designed for energy, immune support, or hydration, providing targeted nutrients to meet those requirements. For example, drinks containing electrolytes and B vitamins might be suitable for rehydration after exercise.

However, it's important to be cautious with vitamin drinks that are high in added sugars or artificial additives. Excessive consumption of sugary vitamin drinks may contribute to increased calorie intake, potentially leading to weight gain and adverse effects on dental health.

Moreover, some vitamin drinks may contain nutrients in amounts that exceed recommended daily allowances. While a balanced diet should ideally provide most essential nutrients, consuming excessive amounts of certain vitamins and minerals, especially fat-soluble vitamins like A, D, E, and K, could lead to adverse health effects.

The best way to obtain necessary vitamins and minerals is through a diverse, balanced diet consisting of fruits, vegetables, whole grains, lean proteins, and healthy fats. Whole foods provide a range of nutrients alongside other beneficial compounds such as fiber, which might not be present in vitamin drinks.

In summary, while vitamin drinks can offer a convenient way to supplement one's nutrient intake, they should not replace a balanced diet. It's important to be mindful of the ingredients and nutritional content in these drinks, opting for options that are low in added sugars and artificial additives. A varied diet with a focus on whole foods remains the foundation for optimal nutrient intake and overall health.

RICE

Rice, a staple food for a significant portion of the world's population, offers several nutritional benefits and versatile uses in various cuisines.

Rice is a rich source of carbohydrates, the body's primary energy source. It provides quick energy due to its high glycemic index, making it an excellent energy booster, especially for individuals engaging in physically demanding activities.

Moreover, rice is gluten-free, making it suitable for individuals with gluten sensitivities or celiac disease. It serves as a staple carbohydrate source in many diets worldwide due to its digestibility and versatility.

Depending on the variety, rice can contain certain essential nutrients. Brown rice, for example, is a whole grain that retains its bran and germ layers, offering more fiber, vitamins, and minerals than white rice. It contains fiber that aids in digestion and helps maintain satiety, potentially aiding in weight management.

Rice also contains small amounts of vitamins and minerals such as B vitamins, manganese, and magnesium. These nutrients play various roles in energy metabolism, bone health, and overall well-being.

While rice provides valuable nutrients and energy, it's important to note that certain processing methods, especially for white rice, remove some of the beneficial components such as fiber and other nutrients present in the bran and germ layers. These processed forms are lower in nutritional value compared to their whole grain counterparts.

Additionally, excessive consumption of refined white rice, especially in the absence of other nutrient-dense foods, might lead to a diet that lacks diversity and adequate essential nutrients.

In conclusion, rice serves as a valuable carbohydrate source and offers some essential nutrients, particularly in its whole grain form. Choosing whole grain varieties such as brown or wild rice provides additional nutritional benefits over refined white rice. When consumed as part of a varied and balanced diet, rice can be an integral component of a healthy eating pattern.

PASTA

Pasta, a staple in various global cuisines, offers several nutritional benefits and culinary versatility. It's a popular carbohydrate source that forms the basis of numerous delicious dishes.

Pasta primarily consists of durum wheat semolina or other grains, providing complex carbohydrates, the body's primary energy source. These carbohydrates supply readily available energy, making pasta a valuable choice for quick fuel, especially for active individuals or athletes.

Whole-grain pasta, made from whole wheat or other whole grains, retains more fiber, vitamins, and minerals compared to refined white pasta. This fiber aids in digestion and contributes to a feeling of fullness, potentially supporting weight management and overall gut health.

Pasta also contains small amounts of essential nutrients such as B vitamins, iron, and magnesium. These nutrients play a role in energy metabolism, red blood cell production, and overall well-being.

While pasta itself is a versatile and valuable food, its nutritional value can vary depending on the ingredients and processing methods used in its production. Whole-grain pasta retains more nutrients and fiber compared to refined white pasta, which undergoes significant processing that removes some beneficial components.

Pairing pasta with nutrient-rich sauces and toppings, such as vegetables, lean proteins, and healthy fats, enhances its overall nutritional value. These additions provide a broader array of nutrients and can transform a simple pasta dish into a balanced and wholesome meal.

However, excessive consumption of refined pasta without accompanying nutrient-dense foods might result in a diet that lacks diversity and adequate essential nutrients.

In summary, pasta is a convenient and versatile carbohydrate source that offers energy and, in its whole-grain form, additional nutritional benefits. Opting for whole-grain varieties can increase the fiber and nutrient content in pasta, making it a more nutritious addition to a balanced diet when combined with other nutrient-rich ingredients. As part of a varied and balanced eating pattern, pasta can be an enjoyable and beneficial component of a healthy meal.

SWEET POTATO

Sweet potatoes, revered for their vibrant color and distinct taste, offer numerous nutritional benefits, making them a popular and versatile vegetable choice.

These tubers are rich in complex carbohydrates, serving as a valuable energy source. Their natural sweetness, attributed to their high fiber content and natural sugars, provides a slower, more sustainable energy release compared to simple carbohydrates, aiding in stabilized blood sugar levels.

One of the standout features of sweet potatoes is their high content of beta-carotene, a precursor to vitamin A. Beta-carotene acts as a powerful antioxidant that supports eye health and overall immune function. The deep orange color of sweet potatoes indicates their high beta-carotene content.

Sweet potatoes also contain other essential vitamins and minerals, such as vitamin C, B vitamins, potassium, and manganese. These nutrients play diverse roles in immune function, energy metabolism, and bone health.

Moreover, sweet potatoes are a good source of dietary fiber. Fiber aids in digestion, promotes a feeling of fullness, and supports gut health. The fiber in sweet potatoes can help regulate bowel movements and contribute to a balanced diet.

Additionally, sweet potatoes offer versatility in cooking. They can be prepared in various ways, from baking and boiling to mashing and roasting. This adaptability makes them a convenient and nutritious addition to a wide range of dishes.

While sweet potatoes provide numerous health benefits, it's important to note that their nutritional value might be influenced by the cooking method and accompanying ingredients. Frying or adding excessive fats and sugars to sweet potatoes might reduce their nutritional profile and potentially negate some of their health advantages.

In conclusion, sweet potatoes are nutrient-dense, offering a range of vitamins, minerals, and fiber. Their rich content of beta-carotene and diverse health benefits make them a valuable addition to a balanced diet when prepared in ways that maintain their nutritional integrity. Incorporating sweet potatoes into various meals can provide both taste and nutrition, contributing to a healthier and well-rounded eating pattern.

CHICKEN

Chicken is a widely consumed and versatile protein source that offers various nutritional benefits, making it a popular choice in many diets worldwide.

Chicken is a rich source of high-quality protein, containing all essential amino acids necessary for muscle repair, growth, and overall bodily functions. Consuming adequate protein from sources like chicken is crucial for building and maintaining muscle mass, supporting a healthy immune system, and aiding in various physiological processes.

Moreover, chicken is relatively low in saturated fat compared to red meats, particularly when the skin is removed. Opting for skinless chicken breast, for example, is an excellent choice for individuals aiming to limit their saturated fat intake, making it a heart-healthier protein option.

Chicken also contains vitamins and minerals such as B vitamins (particularly niacin and B6), phosphorus, and selenium. These nutrients contribute to energy metabolism, nerve function, and the body's antioxidant defense system.

The way chicken is prepared influences its overall nutritional profile. Grilling, baking, or boiling chicken without excessive added fats can help maintain its low-fat content and retain its nutritional value.

However, it's important to note that excessive consumption of chicken, particularly when prepared with high amounts of added fats, breading, or sauces, may increase the intake of saturated fats and calories, potentially impacting health.

In summary, chicken is a lean protein source rich in essential nutrients and amino acids. Selecting lean cuts and preparing chicken in a healthy manner can provide a nutritious addition to a balanced diet. Integrating chicken into meals alongside a variety of vegetables, whole grains, and healthy fats contributes to a well-rounded and nutritious eating pattern.

BEEF

Beef, a commonly consumed red meat, offers various nutritional benefits but should be consumed in moderation due to its specific nutritional profile.

Beef is an excellent source of high-quality protein, delivering all essential amino acids required for muscle maintenance and overall bodily functions. Protein from beef supports muscle growth, repair, and the synthesis of enzymes and hormones within the body.

Additionally, beef is rich in essential nutrients such as iron, zinc, B vitamins (including B12), and selenium. These nutrients play vital roles in red blood cell production, immune function, and overall energy metabolism.

However, beef is also higher in saturated fat compared to other protein sources, which, when consumed in excess, may increase the risk of heart disease and other health issues. Choosing lean cuts of beef and trimming visible fats can help reduce the overall saturated fat content.

Moreover, the method of cooking beef influences its nutritional value. Grilling, broiling, or baking beef without excessive added fats can help maintain its nutrient content while minimizing the intake of unhealthy fats.

It's important to consume beef in moderation and as part of a balanced diet. Opting for leaner cuts and incorporating a variety of protein sources in the diet can help diversify nutrient intake while managing potential health risks associated with high red meat consumption.

In summary, beef provides valuable nutrients such as protein, iron, and B vitamins but should be consumed in moderation due to its higher saturated fat content. Selecting leaner cuts and preparing beef in healthier ways can ensure its nutritional benefits while minimizing potential health risks associated with excessive saturated fat intake. Incorporating beef into a diverse diet alongside other protein sources, vegetables, and whole grains can contribute to a balanced and nutritious eating pattern.

HONEYDEW MELON

Honeydew melon is a refreshing and nutritious fruit that is not typically associated with increasing uric acid levels. In fact, honeydew melon is generally considered a low-purine food, and purines are what break down into uric acid in the body.

For individuals concerned about uric acid levels, it's important to note that honeydew melon contains very low levels of purines, which makes it an unlikely contributor to elevated uric acid.

As a low-purine fruit, honeydew melon is a healthy addition to a balanced diet. It provides essential nutrients, including vitamin C, potassium, and dietary fiber. These nutrients offer a range of health benefits, such as supporting immune function, aiding in digestion, and promoting healthy blood pressure levels.

PAPAYA

Papaya, a tropical fruit, is celebrated for its delicious flavor and diverse health benefits. Rich in essential nutrients, this fruit offers various advantages for overall well-being.

One of the standout components of papaya is its high vitamin C content, crucial for immune function and skin health. It's also a source of antioxidants such as vitamins A and E, helping combat free radicals and potentially reducing the risk of chronic diseases.

The presence of an enzyme called papain in papaya aids in digestion, breaking down proteins and promoting digestive comfort. Additionally, the fruit is a good source of dietary fiber, supporting healthy digestion and regular bowel movements.

Papayas contain beta-carotene, contributing to eye health and potentially reducing the risk of age-related macular degeneration. The high potassium and low sodium content in papaya are beneficial for heart health, helping regulate blood pressure and support proper heart function.

Studies suggest that papaya possesses anti-inflammatory properties, which may help reduce inflammation in the body.

OATS

Oats are a highly nutritious whole grain that offers numerous health benefits and versatility in various culinary applications.

Packed with essential nutrients, oats provide a rich source of complex carbohydrates, supplying a sustained release of energy. The high fiber content in oats, particularly beta-glucans, helps improve digestive health, promotes a feeling of fullness, and assists in maintaining stable blood sugar levels.

Oats are a notable source of various vitamins and minerals, including manganese, phosphorus, magnesium, and B vitamins like thiamine and pantothenic acid. These nutrients play essential roles in energy metabolism, bone health, and overall well-being.

The presence of antioxidants in oats contributes to reducing oxidative stress and inflammation in the body, potentially lowering the risk of chronic diseases. Additionally, oats have been associated with heart health, as their fiber content can help reduce LDL cholesterol levels, aiding in better cardiovascular function.

This versatile grain can be used in various forms, such as oatmeal, granola, or added to baked goods, making it an adaptable and nutritious addition to different recipes.

BANANA

Bananas, one of the most popular and widely consumed fruits globally, offer an array of health benefits and essential nutrients.

Rich in carbohydrates, bananas are an excellent source of quick energy. They contain natural sugars, such as glucose, fructose, and sucrose, providing a convenient and immediate energy boost, making them a great snack before or after physical activities.

Bananas also contain dietary fiber, which aids in digestive health, regulates bowel movements, and promotes a feeling of fullness. They are a good source of vitamin C, an antioxidant that supports immune function and skin health. Additionally, they provide potassium, a crucial mineral for heart health and maintaining proper muscle function.

The fruit is low in sodium and virtually fat-free, making it a healthy and convenient option for various dietary needs. Bananas also contain other essential vitamins and minerals, including vitamin B6 and manganese.

Due to their portability and natural packaging, bananas make for a quick and easy snack that requires no preparation. They can be consumed on their own, added to smoothies, sliced on top of oatmeal or yogurt, or used in baking, offering both taste and nutrition.

Incorporating bananas into your diet provides a natural and nutritious source of essential nutrients and potential health benefits. Whether eaten as a standalone snack or included in various recipes, bananas offer a versatile and healthy addition to a well-rounded diet.

HYGIENE

Juan Vicente Pérez Mora gets a bath every Saturday. A weekly bath ritual, such as the one followed by Juan Vicente Pérez Mora, is pivotal for personal hygiene, skin care, and controlling bacterial accumulation. Regular bathing is a fundamental practice to maintain skin health, eliminate accumulated dirt, sweat, and bacteria, and prevent skin-related issues.

The act of bathing facilitates the removal of surface impurities, reducing the risk of bacterial buildup. It aids in maintaining a healthy skin microbiome and minimizing the potential for skin infections or body odor.

Consistent cleansing through a weekly bath routine supports the elimination of accumulated oils and grime from the skin's surface, contributing to a clearer, refreshed complexion. Moreover, it provides an opportunity for self-examination, allowing individuals to monitor changes in skin health and promptly identify any irregularities or concerns.

Overall, the practice of a weekly bath plays a crucial role in maintaining skin health, minimizing bacterial accumulation, and reducing the risk of skin-related issues. It serves as a fundamental aspect of personal hygiene, ensuring a clean and healthy skin surface.

5 MEALS A DAY

Embracing a dietary routine that involves consuming five meals a day holds several advantages for overall health and well-being. Here's a closer look at the positive impacts of this eating pattern:

Consuming five meals a day supports improved metabolism and sustained energy levels throughout the day. By spacing meals out, individuals can avoid prolonged periods of hunger and maintain a more consistent intake of essential nutrients and energy, promoting a balanced metabolism.

Eating smaller, frequent meals can aid in better portion control and regulate appetite. This approach may reduce the likelihood of overeating during main meals and help in managing weight, as it prevents extreme hunger that can lead to unhealthy snacking or excessive calorie intake.

The distribution of meals across the day allows for a more diverse intake of nutrients, ensuring a balanced diet. It provides an opportunity to incorporate a variety of food groups, offering a broader array of essential vitamins, minerals, and macronutrients necessary for overall health.

Additionally, a routine of five meals a day supports better blood sugar control by preventing significant spikes and drops in blood glucose levels. This balanced approach to eating can be beneficial for individuals who need to manage blood sugar levels, such as those with diabetes or insulin resistance.

Consistency in the five-meal-a-day routine aids in maintaining a more regular eating schedule, reducing cravings, and offering a consistent stream of energy throughout the day. This can lead to improved concentration, better productivity, and sustained energy levels.

In summary, the practice of consuming five meals a day offers multiple health benefits, including improved metabolism, better appetite control, more balanced nutrient intake, and sustained energy levels. This approach to eating supports overall health by providing a steady stream of nutrients, reducing hunger, and improving energy and concentration throughout the day.

ALCOHOL

Moderate alcohol consumption, particularly red wine, has been associated with potential heart health benefits due to compounds like resveratrol and antioxidants present in wine. These elements may positively influence cholesterol levels and reduce inflammation, potentially benefiting cardiovascular health. Some research suggests moderate alcohol intake, like one or two glasses of wine per day, could contribute to improved heart function and reduced risk of heart diseases.

Moreover, the link between moderate alcohol consumption and a reduced risk of certain conditions such as diabetes or dementia has been an area of study. The potential protective effects of alcohol in moderation might have a role in reducing the risk of these health conditions.

These findings suggest that moderate alcohol consumption, particularly red wine, might contribute to overall health and potentially enhance the likelihood of a longer life.

URIC ACID MEDICINE

Juan Vicente Pérez Mora has taken medicine to reduce uric acid in his body. Medications used to lower uric acid levels work by either reducing the production of uric acid in the body or aiding in its elimination. These treatments are typically prescribed to manage conditions like gout, which results from high levels of uric acid.

These medications inhibit enzymes responsible for the production of uric acid. By slowing down this production, they effectively lower the levels of uric acid in the bloodstream. This helps in preventing the formation of uric acid crystals in the joints, reducing the risk of gout attacks and the associated pain and inflammation.

When used in conjunction with lifestyle adjustments, such as dietary changes and increased hydration, these treatments can help manage gout and its symptoms. They play a significant role in reducing the frequency and severity of gout attacks.

GOING TO BED EARLY

Embracing an early bedtime routine offers an array of health benefits and contributes significantly to overall well-being. Here's a focus on the positive impacts of going to bed early:

An early bedtime routine plays a crucial role in supporting physical health, mental acuity, and emotional balance. Getting adequate sleep at an early hour is associated with improved cognitive function, sharper focus, and better overall mood.

Prioritizing an early bedtime creates an opportunity for the body to undergo the essential restorative processes during sleep. It aids in repairing and rejuvenating cells, supporting immune function, and regulating various bodily processes. Adequate sleep is crucial for maintaining optimal health and allowing the body to recuperate from daily stressors.

Moreover, going to bed early promotes better sleep quality, leading to more profound and restful sleep. This contributes to improved energy levels, enhanced mental clarity, and a better ability to tackle tasks and challenges with a refreshed mind.

Consistency in an early bedtime routine helps regulate the body's internal clock, creating a more regular sleep-wake cycle. This results in improved sleep patterns and contributes to better overall health by reducing the risk of sleep-related health issues.

In summary, cultivating a habit of going to bed early is key to maintaining good health and well-being. It enables the body to undergo essential restorative processes during sleep, leading to better overall health, enhanced cognitive function, and improved emotional well-being. An early bedtime routine supports a better quality of sleep, promoting a refreshed and energized start to each day.

47

SOME THOUGHTS

In the journey towards understanding the secrets of longevity, it's important to remember that the path to a long and healthy life is not one-size-fits-all. The insights shared by Juan Vicente Pérez Mora provide a glimpse into his remarkable longevity, but they should be viewed as part of a larger tapestry of factors that contribute to well-being. Here are some thoughts to consider:

Individual Variation: Every person is unique, and what works for one individual may not necessarily work for another. It's crucial to approach longevity with an open mind and a willingness to adapt to your own circumstances and needs.

Flexibility: The daily menu and regime outlined by Mr. Mora can serve as a valuable foundation, but they should not be rigidly adhered to. Life is filled with variables like climate, work, and family responsibilities, and being flexible in your approach is key.

Holistic Well-being: Mr. Mora's insights highlight the importance of not only what you eat but also how you live. Factors like religious practices, sleep habits, and maintaining a calm and relaxed state of mind all play a role in one's health and longevity.

Balanced Diet: The combination of fermented and non-fermented foods, the inclusion of easy-to-digest options, and the emphasis on specific vegetables underscore the significance of a balanced and mindful approach to nutrition.

Cultural and Environmental Influences: Climate, air quality, and local traditions can influence dietary choices and lifestyles. What is suitable for one region may not apply to another. Understanding the impact of your surroundings is essential.

Scientific Basis: Some of Mr. Mora's practices are supported by scientific research, such as the benefits of certain foods like coffee and the effects of religious practices on health. It's important to consider both traditional wisdom and modern scientific knowledge in your approach to longevity.

In the pursuit of a long and healthy life, remember that it's a journey of self-discovery and adaptation. Juan Vicente Pérez Mora's story provides inspiration, but your own path to longevity will be uniquely yours.